MEDICAL CANNABIS

A Guide for Beginners

CYNTHIA NKALA

authorHOUSE®

AuthorHouse™ *UK*
1663 Liberty Drive
Bloomington, IN 47403 USA
www.authorhouse.co.uk
Phone: 0800.197.4150

© *2019 Cynthia Nkala. All rights reserved.*

No part of this book may be reproduced, stored in a retrieval system, or transmitted by any means without the written permission of the author.

The information, ideas, and suggestions in this book are not intended as a substitute for professional medical advice. Before following any suggestions contained in this book, you should consult your personal physician. Neither the author nor the publisher shall be liable or responsible for any loss or damage allegedly arising as a consequence of your use or application of any information or suggestions in this book.

Published by AuthorHouse 02/08/2019

ISBN: 978-1-7283-8449-8 (sc)
ISBN: 978-1-7283-8450-4 (hc)
ISBN: 978-1-7283-8451-1 (e)

Print information available on the last page.

Any people depicted in stock imagery provided by Getty Images are models, and such images are being used for illustrative purposes only.
Certain stock imagery © *Getty Images.*

This book is printed on acid-free paper.

Because of the dynamic nature of the Internet, any web addresses or links contained in this book may have changed since publication and may no longer be valid. The views expressed in this work are solely those of the author and do not necessarily reflect the views of the publisher, and the publisher hereby disclaims any responsibility for them.

CONTENTS

INTRODUCTION... ix
TERMINOLOGY AND ABBREVIATIONS....................... xi

1 THE CANNABIS PLANT

    1.1 Overview... 1
    1.2 Strains Of The Cannabis Plant................................ 2
    1.3 Popular Hybrid Strains Of Cannabis....................... 3
    1.4 Major Cannabinoids And Their Function 4
    1.5 The Difference Between Medical Cannabis
         And Hemp 7
    1.6 Types Of Cannabis Oil 8
    1.7 Legal Status Of Cannabis In The United Kingdom.... 10
    1.8 Current Medical Research For The Use Of
         Cannabis 12

2 CURRENT USES OF CANNABIS
    IN MEDICAL TREATMENT

    2.1 Overview 17
    2.2 Cancer 19

2.3 Multiple Sclerosis 23
2.4 Alzheimer's Disease 26
2.5 Parkinson's Disease... 28
2.6 Stroke 29
2.7 Epileptic Seizures 30
2.8 Arthritis 31
2.9 Irritable Bowel Syndrome 32
2.10 Hepatitis C... 33
2.11 Autoimmune Disease... 34
2.12 Migraine 35
2.13 Metabolism And Digestion 36
2.14 Glaucoma 36
2.15 Stress And Anxiety 37
2.16 Skin Protection.. 38
2.17 Analgesia 39
2.18 Heart Health 40
2.19 Insomnia 41

3   SIDE EFFECTS AND CAUTIONS OF CANNABIS TREATMENT

3.1 Overview.. 43
3.2 Reduced Concentrations 44
3.3 Pregnancy 45
3.4 Psychosis Or Schizophrenia..................................... 46
3.5 Chronic Bronchitis 47
3.6 Risk Of Myocardial Infarction................................. 48

3.7 Risk Of Overdosing Cannabis Oil 49

3.8 Depression And Irritability... 49

4 SOURCES AND STORAGE OF CANNABIS OIL

4.1 How To Get Oil In The Uk..51

4.2 Top Tips When Purchasing Cannabis Online 52

4.3 How To Store Cannabis 55

5 HOW TO MAKE YOUR OWN CANNABIS OIL

5.1 Overview.. 59

5.2 Materials And Equipment Needed 60

5.3 Preparing The Workspace – Step 1......................... 63

5.4 Extracting The Solvent – Step 2 64

5.5 Straining The Mixture – Step 3............................... 65

5.6 Second Soak – Step 4 65

5.7 Separating Cannabis From The Solvent – Step 5 66

5.8 Decarboxylation Of The Oil – Step 6 67

5.9 Adding The Cannabis Mixture To The Carrier Oil.... 68

5.10 Packaging The Cannabis Oil.................................. 69

6 SAFE AND UNSAFE SOLVENTS

6.1 Safe And Unsafe Solvents 71

6.2 Olive Oil – Safe Solvent... 72

6.3 Ethanol And Butane – Safe Solvents 73

6.4 Naphtha And Petroleum Ether – Unsafe Solvents ... 75

7 RECOMMENDED DOSAGES AND DELIVERY ROUTES

7.1 Starting Doses For Beginners 77
7.2 Building Your Tolerance Levels 79
7.3 Dosages For Cancer Patients 81
7.4 Important Lifestyle And Dietary Changes 84
7.5 Maintenance Doses 86

8 HOW TO ADMINISTER CANNABIS OIL

8.1 Overview 87
8.2 Inhalation Method 88
8.3 Oral Method 89
8.4 Rectal/Vaginal Delivery Method 90
8.5 Topical Delivery Method 91
8.6 Sublingual Delivery Method 92

CONCLUSION 93

INTRODUCTION

Have you been wondering 'what cannabis' is, and how it can cure diseases such as cancer? Perhaps you are sceptical about whether cannabis is that effective in the treatment of diseases? Why is it not yet legalised in most countries and particularly in the United Kingdom?

This guide will provide all the basics you might need to know about cannabis. In this guide, the legal status of cannabis is outlined as well as its benefits to human health, and most importantly, how to obtain it and commence treatment. This book is for those who are considering using cannabis as an alternative treatment therapy or for those who need to know more about this wonder herb – cannabis. In this book, you will find background information on the cannabis plant, its varieties and its uses for the treatment of diseases. The guide will also tap into the legal status of medicinal cannabis in the United

Kingdom and instructions on how to make your own cannabis at home.

Like every treatment, cannabis treatment has its pros and cons. However, the positives far outweigh the negatives associated with cannabis. It is therefore advisable to use your personal judgement and make a risk assessment based on your health, whether it's safe to proceed with the treatment or not. Thank you for downloading this book, I hope it will provide valuable information that will help you or your loved ones in their journey to being disease-free individuals.

TERMINOLOGY AND ABBREVIATIONS

<u>Cannabis plant</u> – refers to the plants *Cannabis sativa* and *Cannabis indicia* from which cannabis oil is derived.

<u>THC</u> – stands for 'tetrahydrocannabinol'. This is the principal psychoactive chemical component of cannabis.

<u>Cannabinoid</u> – these are a group of active chemical compounds found in the cannabis plant.

<u>CBD</u> – stands for 'cannabidiol'. It's one of the chemical compounds (cannabinoids) found in the cannabis plant. It is a major phytocannabinoids, accounting for up to 40% of the cannabis plant extract.

<u>CBN</u> – stands for 'cannabinol'. It's another non-psychoactive compound found in the cannabis plant. CBN is a product of oxidised THC.

<u>Cannabis oil</u> – this is defined as a sticky, thick oil made of cannabinoids such as THC and CBD which is extracted

from the cannabis plant. Cannabis oil is also known with various names in today's market, such as marijuana oil, Rick Simpson Oil (RSO) and full extract cannabis oil (FECO).

<u>FECO</u> – stands for 'full extract cannabis oil'. This is a natural concentrate oil derived from the plant *Cannabis sativa*. Natural extraction allows the materials to remain in the oil, hence maintain its healing properties. This oil is also known as Rick Simpson Oil (RSO).

1

THE CANNABIS PLANT

1.1 OVERVIEW

The cannabis plant is defined as the flower and leaves that belong to the Cannabaceae family of plants, which consists of *Cannabis sativa*, *Cannabis Indica* and *Cannabis ruderalis*, (1) although the *ruderalis* is of minor significance. The cannabis plant grows naturally in tropical and temperate climates, but due to high demand, the plant is now being cultivated in most countries using a technology known as indoor hydroponics. The three strains are different in their roles and effects when used for medicinal purposes. The *sativa* strain is the most common of the three, followed by the *Indica* strain, and lastly the *ruderalis* which is not very popular. According to scientists, the cannabis plant is made up of 750 chemicals, amongst which there are different cannabinoids.

1.2 STRAINS OF THE CANNABIS PLANT

Cannabis Indica – this plant is shorter in character and has dense branches, with wider leaves than those of the *sativa* plant. The *Indica* plant grows better if cultivated indoors and has a calming effect on the body and can be effective as a pain relief and alleviating insomnia, therefore it is more effective when taken at bedtime. It's also known for reducing stress and anxiety and can be effective in relaxing the muscles for patients with serious seizures and muscle spasms. (2) The **sativa** strain mostly grows in areas further away from the equator, and it grows best when cultivated outdoors. As opposed to *Indica*, the *sativa* has narrower leaves, loose branches and is much taller. This strain activates energy in the body and increases the state of alertness which leads to more activity. It is also great for optimising focus, hence its effectiveness in alleviating depression.

1.3 POPULAR HYBRID STRAINS OF CANNABIS

'Hybrid strain' refers to a type of strain that has been mixed and consists of two or more different strains. There are top five hybrid strains of *sativa* and *Indica* that are known to produce the best quality cannabis oil. The most popular is **Sour Diesel Strain** – this is invigorating sativa dominant strain which is also known as Sour D or the NY Diesel strain because of its perceived origins in New York City. This strain has a diesel-like aroma with 60% sativa and 40% *Indica*, and its fast acting, delivering energy which can be effective in medical treatments. The Sour D can last for 2-3 hours within the body and is used for treating stress, anxiety and depression.

The second most popular hybrid strain is the **Amnesia Haze Strain**. This strain contains 80% *sativa* and 20% *Indica* and therefore has an energizing effect like Sour D and it's a perfect strain to use if you wish to begin your day with more positivity. This hybrid is stronger and mainly grows in warmer climates, and is perfect for the treatment of depression, fear or migraines. Another hybrid strain is the **Vanilla Kush Strain**, which unlike the other two, is *Indica* dominant, with 80% *Indica* and

20% *sativa*, causing users to be more relaxed and sleepier. This strain originates from the Dutch and it's an indoor or greenhouse type of plant. The Vanilla Kush has a calming effect which makes it the best choice for the treatment of insomnia, stress and depression.

Another popular hybrid strain is the **<u>Orange Hill Special strain</u>**, which is another Dutch hybrid strain that produces 50% *Indica* and 50% *sativa*. This is a balanced hybrid known for its bright orange pistils and citrus flavours which is great for relaxing. The least popular hybrid strain is the **<u>White Rhino</u>**, which is a bushy and stout plant with dark green leaves. The White Rhino is another *Indica* dominant strain with a powerful aroma and contains 14%–20% THC levels which is used in the medical world for the treatment of pain, stress, insomnia and bipolar disorders.

1.4 MAJOR CANNABINOIDS AND THEIR FUNCTION

Cannabinoids are chemical compounds that are found in cannabis plants that determine the quality and type of the cannabis oil produced. There are three different families or categories in which cannabinoids belong to. The first one is the **Phytocannabinoids**, these occur naturally in the *sativa* and *Indica* plants. In this category, there are more than a hundred variations of cannabinoids but only two are active and significant which are **tetrahydrocannabinol (THC) and cannabidiol (CBD)**. The carboxylic acidic properties in cannabis, THCA and CBDA, are decarboxylated into primary cannabinoids known as THC and CBD and these determine the quality and type of oil produced. THC is responsible for the physiological effects of the cannabis plant, stimulating the cells in the human brain, and has a vast number of medicinal properties that will be discussed in the next chapter. The exact concentration of THC in any given cannabis plant depends on the activation of the plant and it ranges between 0.3%–20% by weight. THC is effective in our bodies because it connects with receptor systems in the human body, the endocannabinoid system. The second primary cannabinoid is cannabidiol (CBD) and its properties are the opposite to that of THC. CBD is completely non-pyscho-active, is more relaxing in nature and has properties which include anti-inflammatory and anti-oxidant effects. The actual concentration of CBD in any cannabis plant varies, ranging between 0.6%–1%, and this percentage expresses how much CBD is in the cannabis compared to other compounds that make up the plant.

Another family of cannabinoids is the **endocannabinoids.** These are created from the human body and are the lipids and glands that the body has without any ingestion of the cannabis plant. The endocannabinoid system (ECS) is defined as a group of cannabinoid receptors within the brain and nervous system that is responsible for a variety of physiological changes such as pain sensation, appetite, mood and memory. Just like THC, CBD interacts with endocannabinoids and activates the body's natural response to pain, anxiety and stress within the nervous system.

The third family of cannabinoids is the **synthetic cannabinoids**, which are man-made in the laboratory, but they structurally resemble the phytocannabinoids and the endocannabinoids and they have similar biological mechanisms. Another cannabinoid, which is of minor significance, is *cannabinol (CBN)*. This cannabinoid is not produced by the plant, but it is formed by THC breakdown due to poor storage or degradation. The THC is then oxidised to create CBN which has no medicinal properties, and neither is it strong.

1.5 THE DIFFERENCE BETWEEN MEDICAL CANNABIS AND HEMP

According to the North American Industrial Hemp Council, if the cannabis plant has a THC content less than 0.5%, then it is classified as hemp. In simpler terms, hemp is another type of cannabis that has been stripped of many cannabinoids and is widely available on the market for industrial and medicinal uses. In most countries, hemp is cultivated for industrial purposes with a minimum percentage of THC. Due to the THC being stripped from the plant, the cultivated hemp is very different to the original – it is thinner and therefore easy to harvest. As opposed to medicinal cannabis, hemp has no effect as a recreational drug, and therefore smoking hemp causes a headache, not a 'high'.

Hemp is used as a main ingredient in the production of oil paints, cosmetics and food supplements and therefore has a wide variety of industrial uses. The world's largest producer of industrial hemp is France, producing more than 70% of the world output, with China being the second largest producer. However, not all types of hemp are authorised for cultivation in Europe. Participating countries are only allowed to grow varieties that have been certified by the European Union. If you intend to grow hemp in the United Kingdom, you will need to apply for cultivation licences from the Home Office under the Misuse of Drugs Act 1971.

1.6 TYPES OF CANNABIS OIL

The cannabis oil which is derived from the cannabis plant, has been classified into four types. The first is **_Medical Marijuana Oil_**; this oil has the highest concentration of THC because it is produced from female cannabis plants or from the flowers. It has THC concentration levels between 70–90% and relatively low levels of CBD which are less than 5%. Higher THC levels makes it suitable for medicinal purposes. This type of oil is produced using liquid butane as a solvent for extraction, which is why it is sometimes referred to as Marijuana Butane Honey Oil. The second type of oil is **_Medical Cannabis Oil_**, which is like the above, but is produced from the whole plant – parts of it from the marijuana section of the plant and from the hemp part. The THC concentration levels in this oil are slightly lower than in Marijuana Oil and it ranges between 50–60% whilst the CBD concentrations remain lower than 5%. However, this type of oil is still an excellent choice for the treatment of diseases.

The third type of oil is **_High CBD Oil_**, also known as hemp oil. However, hemp is stronger than the industrial one and is effective in medical uses because of the high CBD levels which then balance off with the THC levels in the human body. This oil consists of approximately 40% THC levels and a relatively higher level of CBD ranging between 10–15%. This type of hemp is different because it carries high THC levels and therefore is appropriate for the treatment of diseases. The seeds of hemp are useful and can be used in cosmetic production. They are also nutritious and produce fatty acids such as omega 3 and omega 6, which are essential in the maintenance of cardiac health.

The fourth type of oil is the most common one known as **_Rick Simpson Cannabis Oil_**. This was named after a former Canadian cancer patient who pioneered the production of cannabis oil using non-petroleum solvents. This type of oil is made with organic solvents such as olive oil. It's also easy to make – most patients can make their own oil at home. Rick Simpson oil is high in THC concentration, but also contains CBD properties and hence it is effective in the treatment of diseases, and mostly popular in cancer patients. There is a step-by-step guide on how to make this type of oil at home that will be outlined in Chapter 4.

1.7 LEGAL STATUS OF CANNABIS IN THE UNITED KINGDOM

Cannabis is classified as a class B drug in the United Kingdom, which means it's illegal to be found in possession of it or selling the drug. The herb became first illegal in 1928 following the International Drugs Convention in Geneva when an Egyptian delegate convinced everyone that cannabis was a threat to society. In 1971, the UK government then passed the Misuse of Drugs Act, which classified cannabis into a class B drug, meaning breaking this rule will attract penalties. The positive thing with this act is that it allowed research on medical cannabis. However, there has been growing awareness and campaign on cannabis which led to the European

Economic Community (EEC) Directive in 1993, which allowed farmers to grow the plant with minimal contents of THC under the licence of the relative authority.

There has been a growing campaign by members of parliament in the United Kingdom to legalise cannabis. Ministers argue that with cannabis being the most used illegal drug in the country, it's costing huge amounts of money to the taxpayer. According to the Daily News, UK, the illegality of cannabis is costing one billion pounds per year to the taxpayer and approximately 6.7% of the total population are using it every year. The campaign by members of parliament is not aimed at the recreational effects of the drug but on its magnificent uses as a treatment drug. The UK government has been urged to follow other countries like the USA and legalise cannabis, which has led to the production of a legalised cannabis drug known as Sativex, which is currently available on the NHS for MS patients only. The drug Sativex, manufactured by GW Pharmaceuticals, is expensive, costing the NHS a minimum of £375.00 for each patient supply. The reason for the high cost of this drug is attributed to the legal status of cannabis, making it expensive to obtain authorisation, and the cost of research and development.

Although medical cannabis (with CBD only), has been legalised to be manufactured by authorised manufacturers in the UK, THC remains a class B drug. Doctors can prescribe cannabis medicines but unfortunately, they can't prescribe raw cannabis for medicine. Across the world, most countries are warming up to this drug, with most states legalising it in the USA and countries where most research is conducted. Rules regarding cannabis differ for each country, therefore if travelling from one country to another, get a valid medical cannabis card if it applies to your country. This card authorises you to be in possession of your cannabis medicines and saves you the hassle of questioning by police.

1.8 CURRENT MEDICAL RESEARCH FOR THE USE OF CANNABIS

The medical world is conducting a vast amount of research globally, on the use cannabis as a treatment option. Ongoing research conducted at one of the biggest centres for medical research in California, the Medicinal

Cannabis Research, University of California, USA. This institution aims at co-ordinating rigorous scientific studies that assess the safety and effectiveness of cannabis compounds in treating various medical conditions.

Israel is one of the top countries exploring the effects of cannabis as a medical treatment, and it has the best scientific cannabis researchers. Israel is amongst the first countries that legalised medical cannabis, and hence enabled them to undertake a lot of clinical research funded by the Israeli government. One of the popular Israeli researchers, Raphael Mechoulam, who began his research back in the 1960s, has been very successful in his research. Raphael was able to synthesise cannabinoids, which made way for pharmaceutical research and clinical trials on the effects of these cannabinoids.

Back home in the UK, despite cannabis not yet being legalised, some scientific research is being conducted on the effectiveness of cannabis treatment. GW Pharmaceuticals, a UK-based company that manufactures drugs, conducted a study in 2016 on the effects of cannabis on Davet's Syndrome, which is a rare type of epilepsy that is normally diagnosed in children and young adults. The research produced positive results and proved that cannabis can deliver a significant reduction in seizures, thereby improving the quality of life for patients diagnosed with Davet's Syndrome.

The National Health Service (NHS) has also conducted a fair amount of research to establish the effectiveness of cannabis treatments. Over the past decade, the NHS explored the effects of cannabis on patients diagnosed with multiple sclerosis (MS), in a study which was funded by the Medical Research Council, UK. The result of this research was successful, and it enabled the NHS to acquire the cannabis-based medication, Sativex, for MS patients. The NHS also investigated the effectiveness of cannabis as an analgesic, aimed at monitoring the effects of cannabinoids on post-operative pain. The research results were positive and proved that cannabis has properties that can significantly reduce the pain after surgery.

More recently, during the summer of 2017, Britain has opened its first official weed research facility for medical cannabis. This is positive news in the medical cannabis world and promises a bright and successful future for all health care facilities and the public in general. In a quest to find treatment for cancer diseases, this new facility will explore and conduct a thorough examination of the use of THC as a treatment for cancer. The process will involve a lot of clinical trials and research into the medicinal applications of different cannabinoids, with the aim of producing a licenced portfolio of licenced cannabis-based medications soon. The regulatory body that governs these medicines, known as the Medicines and Healthcare Products Regulatory Agency (MHRA), is in support of this initiative and confirms that cannabinoids have a restoring, correcting and modifying effect on physiological functions of the human body.

Although there is a significant amount of research done on cannabis treatment, the world has not yet fully accepted and embraced it as a medicinal drug which can be made available to the public. The hindrance to this acceptance is the lack of clinical trials that can pave the way for its acceptance and prove its effectiveness as a medicinal drug. Most of the research which has been done is laboratory-based, meaning it's been carried out on animals prior to human trialling. The reason for the slow pace in clinical trials is the government position on the use of cannabis. The restrictions made by governments make it very difficult for clinical researchers to progress to the next level. If governments lift the ban on medical cannabis, there is a promising future in the healthcare industry.

2

CURRENT USES OF CANNABIS IN MEDICAL TREATMENT

2.1 OVERVIEW

Cannabis has been defined as the wonder drug by many, due to its ability to treat a wide spectrum of diseases. Over the years, cannabis has been used to treat a variety of diseases and their symptoms, which will be further elaborated in this chapter. The diseases discussed in this chapter are not an exhaustive list but an overview of the major conditions where cannabis herb treatment has been a success. Apart from the treatment of diseases, cannabis has been associated with developing sharp brains, hence it was recommended for military men and intellect advisors.

Although being 'high' affects the short-term memory, cannabis has been claimed to improve the creativity of the mind, thereby enabling users to achieve better results in examinations and able to create new ideas.

Cannabis has also been used to help patients addicted to opiate analgesia such as morphine. There have been suggestions that taking cannabis oil will enable patients to safely withdraw from opiate drugs, ensuring a steady rehabilitation. Some have used cannabis for weight loss, although there is not enough evidence to prove its effectiveness. Those who have used cannabis oil to reduce weight have claimed it to be effective, depending on the type of strain chosen. THC cannabinoids are known to increase appetite and hence will result in weight gain, whilst CBD suppresses the appetite. Therefore, if you intend to use cannabis for weight loss, you will need a strain which has higher concentrations of CBD and low levels of THC. These are some of the non-medical uses of cannabis. However, the rest of this chapter will focus on the medicinal effects of cannabinoids in the treatment of diseases such as cancer, multiple sclerosis and Parkinson's, just to mention a few.

2.2 CANCER

One of the major and exciting uses of the cannabis plant is the ability to treat cancer. Cancer is one of the major killers in the western world. Therefore, any form of therapy that can destroy this disease is welcomed with hope. Researchers have done a lot of work in trying to establish the effectiveness of cannabinoids on cancer cells. The results of all the studies done have proved that cannabis has the potential to be a catalyst in the eradication of cancer as a disease. According to a discovery published in the Journal Molecular Therapeutics, cannabinoids prevent the spread of cancer by disabling a gene known as id-1. This gene is the main culprit in the spreading of cancer because it acts as a catalyst in spreading the tumour cells, replicating copies of itself and thereby spreading the disease throughout the body. Cannabis' ability to reduce these id-1 genes in the body is of major interest to studies and it gives them a ray of hope. The id-1-focused research was conducted at the California Pacific Medical Centre in San Francisco back in 2007. This research studied breast cancer cells in the laboratory that had high levels of id-1, which were treated with cannabinoids. A positive outcome was achieved, with breast cancer cells displaying a reduced id-1 expression and less aggressive tumour cells.

Apart from disabling id-1 genes, cannabinoids have some anti-tumour effects in cancer cells in many ways, which includes inducing cell death, prohibiting cell growth, stopping tumour invasion and blocking metastasis. Following research, there are promising results on anti-cancer treatment for cancers such as breast cancer, liver cancer and leukaemia, just to mention a few. Another exciting discovery by scientists is that cannabinoids encourage cytosis, which is the programmed cell death of cancer cells by blocking the production of the tumour's blood vessels. Apart from a direct attack on cancer, cannabinoids also help in treating symptoms of the disease, alleviating pain, nausea and anxiety. Anxiety is one of the unpleasant effects in patients diagnosed with cancer, as they are uncertain if they will win the battle or not. The Harvard University Medical School conducted a study which drew the conclusion that cannabinoids have the ability to improve the mood by reducing anxiety. However, for cannabis to effectively attack anxiety, it should be taken moderately – otherwise if taken in larger doses, it might have the opposite effect and increase paranoia.

Another great effect of cannabis is during chemotherapy treatment, where it can reduce the side effects of chemotherapy, with patients appreciating a reduction in pain, nausea and increased appetite. Although chemotherapy and radiotherapy are both effective in the destruction of cancer cells, these treatments come with awful side effects. Therefore, if not using cannabis as your main treatment, you can use it to control the side effects of chemotherapy and radiotherapy, following approval from your doctors. It is important to be able to manage these side effects as they can lead to other health complications and significantly reduce the quality of life. Although some patients have taken a leap of faith in treating cancer with cannabinoids only, without other conventional treatments, research has proved that combining cannabis with these treatments is more effective. This theory has been supported by laboratory experiments which tested the combination of cannabinoids with other chemotherapy drugs such as gemcitabine and temozolomide. The results of these experiments were positive; however, the choice still rests with everyone depending on what would be the best approach, based on the reliability of the medical advice they get.

In as much as cannabinoids have proven to be effective in the treatment of cancer, unfortunately it's not all 100% good news. Cannabinoids also present a negative impact on the human body and unwanted side effects. Just like chemotherapy, high doses of THC can destroy cancer cells, but destroy crucial blood vessels in the process. However, this must not discourage those who wish to try cannabis treatment, because the positives outweigh the negatives by far, and whatever treatment option you choose, there will be always pros and cons. These negative effects of cannabinoids depend on the dosages and levels of the cannabinoid receptors on the cancer cells. Research has claimed that the cannabinoid receptor known as CB2 interferes with the ability of the immune system to destroy cancer cells, hence producing an overall negative outcome. Another disadvantage of cannabis on cancer cells is that it can develop a resistance to cannabinoids due to constant use, and as a result, cancer cells will grow again. However, a solution was developed to counteract this effect, known as ALK. This system works by blocking a certain molecular pathway that abolishes the resistance to the THC treatment of tumour cells. Although there are some disadvantages to using cannabis in treatment, it remains a crucial herb in alternative therapies for cancer diseases.

2.3 MULTIPLE SCLEROSIS

Cannabis had a breakthrough in the management and treatment of symptoms of multiple sclerosis, commonly known as MS. Multiple sclerosis is defined as an inflammatory and autoimmune degenerative disease of the central nervous system that affects the brain, spinal cord and the optic nerve. This disease affects millions of people around the world and unfortunately no cure has been found for it yet. The symptoms of MS include pain, incontinence, cognitive decline and fatigue, and all these negatively impact the quality of life for diagnosed patients.

Across the world, many MS patients have attempted cannabis treatment, and it has proven to be effective in relieving pain, gastrointestinal distress, muscle spasms and paralysis amongst MS sufferers. A study conducted in the United Kingdom confirmed there is a significant number of MS patients who are using cannabinoids for symptoms relief. About 14–18% of patients in the case study reported less pain and spasms. Therefore, cannabis treatment can be used as a complementary therapy for MS, in addition to the powerful drugs which are aimed at slowing the disease progression, managing symptoms and speeding up recovery from attacks.

Jody Corey, a cannabis researcher, conducted a study on the impact of cannabis on MS sufferers, particularly focusing on the painful contractions of their muscles. The results of this study were published in the Canadian Medical Association Journal and claimed that after a few days of using cannabinoids, patients reported a significant reduction in pain and muscle spasms. In this study of 30 MS patients, Jody found that THC cannabinoids bind the receptors in the nerves and muscles to achieve pain reduction and reduced muscle spasms. Both the THC and CBD cannabinoids act as effective analgesics by engaging pain receptors in the body, destroying the pain signals sent by the nerve cells to provide much-needed pain relief.

Muscle spasms and stiffness negatively impact the quality of life for patients living with multiple sclerosis. By reducing muscle stiffness and spasms, cannabis therefore improves their quality of life. Evidence taken from the studies from two universities, the University of Plymouth, UK, in 2012 and Tel Aviv University in Israel have both revealed that cannabis was twice as effective at relieving muscle spasms and stiffness as compared to the placebo used. Following a study period of twelve weeks, both universities reported a significant reduction in spasticity amongst MS patients, as compared to their counterparts on the placebo. Spasticity is another symptom for MS patients whereby they have uncontrollable muscle stiffness and twitching.

Another way in which cannabis is helpful in the relief of MS symptoms is its ability to protect the human brain from inflammation. Inflammation is a major challenge for MS patients, and this is due to the activation of immune cells, which then releases pro-inflammatory proteins known as cytokines, which are responsible for causing inflammation in the brain. The CBD and THC cannabinoids deactivate the immune system and prohibit this violent attack on the central nervous system. Cannabinoids contain compounds which are anti-oxidants, and this arms them with the neuro-properties that can fight inflammation. Another benefit of using cannabis in managing MS is that it helps with digestion, because THC is an appetite stimulant – therefore, it triggers the release of hunger hormones to kick start the metabolism, thereby reducing gastrointestinal inflammation.

Insomnia is another symptom that reduces the quality of life for MS sufferers. Cannabis can therefore act as a sleeping tablet, enabling patients to sleep faster and for longer periods. Cannabinoids will attack the pain and insomnia, enabling the patients to have a deep sleep which is essential for the body to repair itself. Another unpleasant symptom for MS is blurry vision, uncontrollable eye movements and inflammation of the optical nerve. If these symptoms are not managed, patients can have episodes of blindness. Therefore, it is essential to resolve it as soon as possible. Studies have proven that cannabinoids are effective in protecting the eyes by reducing inflammation of the optic nerve and hence reducing these awful effects on the optical nerve.

2.4 ALZHEIMER'S DISEASE

Dementia is one of the most common diseases in the ageing population in the UK, and it affects approximately 47.5 million people across the world. Alzheimer's disease is the most common type of dementia, which causes a decline in memory, thinking and behaviour and it has a massive negative impact on the quality of life of diagnosed patients. According to the World Health Organisation

(WHO), dementia is now the leading cause of death in England and Wales, overtaking heart disease. A vast amount of research has been conducted to prove the effectiveness of cannabis on dementia, and promising results have been achieved. Alzheimer's disease causes inflammation of the brain, which then creates a plaque of amyloid that kills the brain cells. In a study led by Kim Janda of the Scripps Research Institute, published in the journal Molecular Pharmaceuticals (2006), it was reported that THC slows down the formation of amyloid plaques by blocking the enzyme in the brain that produces these plaques. Another study that proved the same results has been conducted at the Roskamp Institute in Florida, published by the Molecular and Cellular Neuro Science Journal, claiming that cannabinoids clear the prevalence of beta-amyloid plaque in the brain and hence slows down the progression of the disease.

CBD cannabinoids have some neuroprotective antioxidant properties that are essential in the treatment of Alzheimer's disease. The build-up of the amyloid plaques in the brain causes neurotoxicity, which accelerates cell death. Research has claimed that CBD reduces brain cell death by reducing neurotoxicity caused by plaques – they stimulate cell growth and play a vital role in the growth of neural tissue in the hippocampus, an area on the brain associated with memory. One of the more compelling arguments for the use of medicinal cannabis is its ability to alleviate other symptoms of Alzheimer's such as loss of appetite, weight loss and agitation, thereby allowing patients to live happier and, most importantly, functional lives. The improved quality of life that cannabis offers to Alzheimer patients has encouraged researchers to focus more on the clinical research of its effectiveness. Although these findings are still preliminary, researchers are hoping more clinical research on Alzheimer's disease.

2.5 PARKINSON'S DISEASE

Researchers and scientists began to show interest on Parkinson's disease following numerous testimonies on social media in relation to the effectiveness of cannabis on reducing tremors that affect diagnosed patients. Parkinson's disease is defined as a degenerative disorder of the central nervous system that mainly affects the motor system. Parkinson's disease is caused by a reduction of the chemical dopamine in the body, which then lead to factories in the human body to die. Dopamine helps muscles to move smoothly, and therefore insufficient levels or unavailability of this chemical can cause tremors. According to a recent study from Israeli researchers, cannabinoids can significantly reduce pain and tremor for Parkinson's disease patients. What is particularly interesting about the results of this research is that cannabis can significantly improve fine motor skills for Parkinson's disease patients. Thanks to the Israeli researchers for conducting this study, it gives hope to the patients for an improved quality of life.

2.6 STROKE

Over the past years, patients diagnosed with stroke have attempted to treat the effects of stroke using cannabis, and success has been achieved in protecting the brain following a stroke. A stroke is a serious life-threatening medical condition that occurs when the blood supply to part of the brain is cut off. This will result in the brain cells being deprived of oxygen and dying, causing some physical disability to the patient. According to pre-clinical research which was conducted at the University of Nottingham in the UK, cannabinoids can heal the brain following a concussion and other traumatic injury and protect the brain from damage caused by stroke. Please note, STROKE IS A MEDICAL EMERGENCY – if you think you have symptoms of stroke, call 999 immediately. Cannabis does not treat a stroke, but it helps as part of the rehabilitation process, and to prevent it from reoccurring.

2.7 EPILEPTIC SEIZURES

There has been news circulating on the media on the positive effects of cannabis on Dravet's Syndrome, which is a rare type of epileptic seizure that mainly affects children and young adults. An epileptic seizure is a brief episode of jerking and uncontrollable movements caused by extra activities in the brain. Research is ongoing to explore the effectiveness of cannabis on Dravet's syndrome, and GW Pharmaceuticals (UK) has recently announced positive results on the phase (iii) trial of the cannabinoid-based epilepsy drug known as Epidiolex. This drug has presented a significant reduction in the frequency of convulsive seizures in diagnosed children. CBD cannabinoids control the seizures by binding the cells that are responsible for controlling excitability and regulating relaxation. Some American scientists and doctors have recommended cannabis treatment for epilepsy, claiming that cannabinoids interact with the brain cells to calm excessive activities in the brain that cause these seizures. This research on epilepsy is promising, and there is hope for cure of Dravet's syndrome, improving the quality of life for patients.

2.8 ARTHRITIS

The cannabis plant is also helpful in alleviating the pain in arthritis patients. Arthritis is a common condition that causes pain and inflammation of the joints, the two most common types being osteoarthritis and rheumatoid arthritis. Researchers have discovered that cannabis relieves arthritis by reducing inflammation and pain and promoting sleep, which is essential for the body to heal. In one of the studies done, trial patients were given Sativex, which is a cannabis-based analgesia and great results were achieved. After a two-week trial, patients on Sativex reported a significant reduction in pain and improved sleep as compared to the patients on the placebo. Some arthritic patients prefer to ingest the cannabis as tea, and this high-CBD tea has positive reviews regarding its effectiveness. The other advantage of CBD tea is that it is cost effective and does not cause the patients to feel side effects such as being 'high' or 'dopey'.

2.9 IRRITABLE BOWEL SYNDROME

Irritable bowel syndrome, commonly known as IBS, is a disorder that affects the large intestine, particularly the colon, causing some abdominal cramping, bloating, gas, pain and constipation. The cannabis herb has been effective in relieving the symptoms of Crohn's disease and ulcerative colitis which are both irritable bowel diseases. According to a study conducted at the University of Nottingham in 2010, cannabinoids interact efficiently with human body cells, playing a vital role in the gut functions and immune response. The human body produces its own cannabinoids, which increase the permeability of the intestines, therefore allowing bacteria into the gut. Cannabinoids from the plant will then block the human cannabinoids, preventing this permeability, and therefore the intestine cells are bonded together. In a study published in the Journal of Pharmacology and Experimental Therapeutics, it was proved that cannabis can be effective in the management and treatment of IBS. Cannabis was trialled on patients with Crohn's disease, and ten out of eleven patients responded well to treatment presenting reduced symptoms. Even more impressive was that five of those patients were in complete remission.

2.10 HEPATITIS C

Cannabis has been used to lessen the side effects that patients suffer following hepatitis C treatment. Hepatitis C is a viral infection of the liver that causes inflammation and fibrosis. Cannabinoids do not treat the hepatitis c virus but do reduce the effects of its harsh side effects such as fatigue, loss of appetite, nausea and muscle aches. These side effects can be so bad that some patients are unable to cope and therefore will not complete their treatment regime. This is where cannabinoids come in, to counteract the negative side effects of hepatitis C medications and make it more tolerable. This was proven following a study published in the European Journal of Gastroenterology and Herpetology in 2006, where 86% of patients who used cannabis whilst on hepatitis C treatment successfully completed their treatment as compared to only 29% of non-cannabis users who completed their treatment. Although cannabis does not treat hepatitis C, this study showed that cannabis might still have a small but significant impact on the hepatitis C itself. This was proven by the results of 54% of patients who were on both hepatitis C treatment and cannabis, and managed to get their viral levels low, compared to the 8% who did not use cannabis and struggled to lower their viral levels. It is therefore advisable to try cannabis when struggling with the side effects of hepatitis C treatment.

2.11 AUTOIMMUNE DISEASE

An autoimmune disease is a condition whereby the body's immune system attacks itself by mistake, instead of protecting the body from diseases and infection. There are more than 80 types of autoimmune diseases and all of them have similar symptoms which makes them difficult to diagnose. The most common autoimmune disease includes rheumatoid arthritis, systematic lupus erythematosus, psoriasis and inflammatory bowel disease. The primary goal in treating autoimmune diseases is to reduce inflammation, and that's where cannabinoids come in. Research has been conducted to establish the effectiveness of cannabis on the disease lupus erythematosus, which affects the skin, joints, kidneys and other organs. The chemicals in cannabinoids have a calming effect on the immune system, because of their ability to fight inflammation, which is a major symptom of autoimmune diseases. Apart from inflammation, cannabinoids can fight pain and nausea, which can be a challenge to patients diagnosed with lupus and other autoimmune diseases.

2.12 MIGRAINE

Another discovery made by researchers on cannabis is the ability to treat migraines. A migraine is a moderate to severe headache felt as a throbbing pain on one side of the head, with symptoms such as nausea, vomiting and increased sensitivity to light and sound. There have been numerous testimonies from patients who used cannabis to treat their migraine, reporting some tremendous results. Although not much clinical evidence has been pursued in relation to the effects of cannabis on migraine, there are reports from patients that it is very helpful in the management of migraine. Unfortunately, cannabis has not yet licenced in the UK, therefore doctors cannot prescribe it. However, some migraine patients in the UK have used Charlotte Web Hemp Extract Oil, which is available to purchase online, and they can ship internationally.

Please be advised, it is very important to make your own assessment before purchasing any cannabis and ensure that the supplier is genuine and credible.

2.13 METABOLISM AND DIGESTION

Cannabinoids have been found to be helpful for the metabolism, enabling weight loss. The American Journal of Medicine published a study that showed that people who use cannabis are not only thinner but have healthier metabolisms and sugar reactions. This case study analysed data from 4500 adult Americans, of which 570 used cannabis as treatment, and explored how the bodies of cannabis users responded to the consumption of sugars. This study included a thorough assessment of their insulin levels during a nine-hour fasting period and the time they were not fasting. The results of the research showed that in those patients using cannabis, their bodies could break down sugars in a healthier way, promoting metabolism.

2.14 GLAUCOMA

Cannabis has been used to treat glaucoma, which is an eye condition where the optic nerve, which connects the eye to the brain, becomes damaged (NHS). Glaucoma can lead to loss of vision, due to the pressure inside the eye not draining properly. A study conducted by Nucci et al. (2008) concluded that CBD and THC cannabinoids work in the body like the endocannabinoid system, decreasing the intraocular pressure that leads to glaucoma. Cannabinoids have also been useful in the treatment of macular degeneration, which is a painless eye condition that causes loss of central vision, making it difficult to read, differentiate colours or recognise faces. According to a pre-clinical study which was conducted in the eye research laboratory, cannabinoids were able to treat rats with eye problems, and they experienced less damage to their photoreceptors as compared to untreated rats. The treatment was effective because of the anti-oxidant properties of cannabinoids which help reduce pro-angiogenic factors, hence treating macular degeneration. However, it is important to consult your optician before using cannabis oil for eye treatment.

2.15 STRESS AND ANXIETY

Over many years, cannabis has been used as a stress reliever and to reduce emotional trauma. In an Israeli study published in the Psych-Neuroendocrinology Journal (2013), cannabinoids were found to be effective in the treatment and prevention of stress-induced impairments. Cannabinoids achieved this result because THC minimises stress receptors in the hippocampus and basolateral amygdala, thereby stimulating pleasure hormones. In a recent study published in 2015, it was stated that THC does the same function as the human endocannabinoid system which regulates anxiety in the body. Because of these similar characteristics, both THC and endocannabinoids have the same effect in reducing stress and anxiety because they act in the same pathway. Military veterans have been advised to use cannabis, especially those suffering from PTSD (post-traumatic stress disorder) and have had their symptoms relieved and continued to live peaceful lives.

2.16 SKIN PROTECTION

One of the popular industrial uses of cannabis is in the cosmetics sector, being used as hemp oil to manufacture skin creams, oils and lotions. CBD oil can protect the skin from diseases and infections because it contains omega 3 and omega-6 fatty acids, which are very effective in maintaining a healthy skin and giving it a glowing look. Cannabinoids improve the skin appearance by removing dead skin and oils, promoting the production of healthy new cells to replace dead ones. Researchers have reported that due to the cannabis' high levels of anti-oxidant properties, cannabinoids fight against cell damage, thus preventing ageing signs such as wrinkles, blemishes and skin spots. Apart from maintaining skin appearances, cannabinoids treat chronic skin diseases such as psoriasis, acne, eczema and rosacea. This is because cannabinoids promote the production of lipids which protect the skin by giving it a break from attack by these diseases.

2.17 ANALGESIA

In every disease or condition treated with cannabis, the analgesic effect has been one of its popular characteristics. In a study conducted by a Canadian researcher (2010), a sample of 23 adults diagnosed with neuropathic pain resulting from surgery and trauma were treated with different doses of cannabis oil. The results of this study showed that patients who took cannabis three times a day reported less pain as compared to the patients who took it twice a day. The analgesic effect of cannabinoids is due to them being an effective neural transmitter in the body's pain pathways and therefore achieving pain reduction. Cannabinoids work in collaboration with the endocannabinoids of the human body which control pain, improving the functionality of reducing neuropathic and chronic pains.

2.18 HEART HEALTH

The heart is one of the most important organs of the body. Therefore, it is very important to ensure that the heart is in good health. There are several heart-related diseases, most of them being life-threatening, resulting in a huge number of deaths. Researchers have claimed that cannabinoids have a positive effect on the cardiovascular system, strengthen the heart muscles and reduce cholesterol levels. Cannabis enhances the heart health because of its anti-oxidant properties that are very beneficial in the cell reinforcement process of the heart muscle. Evidence gathered from the British Animal Study, published in the Pharmacological Research Journal (2014), suggested that cannabinoids help to widen and relax the blood vessels, therefore reducing blood pressure, improving circulation and protecting the heart from heart attack and stroke.

2.19 INSOMNIA

Insomnia is a common symptom of several diseases and can have a negative impact on the quality of life. Sleep is essential for the body to heal; therefore, for any form of treatment to be effective, it should be accompanied by a healthy sleeping pattern. Cannabinoids have had a calming effect and anti-anxiety properties help improve sleep breathing problems and reduce sleep interruptions as well. According to the journal Frontiers in Psychiatry Sleep Disorder (2013), cannabinoids help to create a variety of focal sensory systems and direct neurotransmitter discharges, which leads to increased pleasure, therefore leading to an improved sleep. Because of this effect, it is worth trying cannabinoids as a sleeping tablet to enhance the recovery of the body from disease.

3

SIDE EFFECTS AND CAUTIONS OF CANNABIS TREATMENT

3.1 OVERVIEW

Like any other medications and treatments, cannabis treatment has its own side effects and contra-indications that patients need to be aware of. These side effects include psychosis, chronic bronchitis and a low risk of myocardial infarction. This chapter will explore the side effects and cautions that patients need to be aware of when undertaking cannabis treatment.

3.2 REDUCED CONCENTRATIONS

The most common side effect of cannabis is the alteration of concentration levels. Cannabis can affect the memory, ability to think properly, and reduce concentration levels. Decreased concentration levels can have an impact on the ability to do certain tasks which require high levels of concentration and can also affect the ability to work. It is advised not to take cannabis together with medications such as anti-depressants, strong analgesics and muscle relaxers, because medications can cause increased drowsiness and fatigue, therefore negatively affecting the levels of concentration. If you must work during your cannabis treatment, it is recommended to take high doses of cannabis at bedtime rather than in the morning, so that the negative effects do not hinder your daily activities. It is also not advisable to drive if you have taken cannabis oil within the last six hours, as your concentration levels will be impaired and can result in fatal road accidents. Driving under the influence of any drugs is a crime, and if found with cannabis in your blood it might land you in jail.

3.3 PREGNANCY

There have been some controversial debates around the use of cannabis during pregnancy. The three major arguments against the use of cannabis during pregnancy are (i) growth issues such as low birth weight, (ii) implications on foetal brain development, and (iii) high risk of premature birth. Several pieces of research have been conducted in New Zealand and Australia on the effects of cannabis on pregnancy. The results of these studies proved that parents who used cannabis during pregnancy had a greater probability of pre-term delivery and significant chances of SIDS (sudden infant death syndrome). However, not everyone agrees with the above research findings, and some researchers argue that cannabis does not have adverse effects on the unborn child. In a study conducted by a Jamaican researcher, Dr Melanie Dreher and her team, it was shown that there is no difference on the babies born from parents who took cannabis whilst pregnant, and babies where cannabis was not involved. Although Dr Melanie Dreher's research suggests zero effect of cannabis on the foetus, there is not enough research to prove that the herb is safe during pregnancy. For the sake of protecting the unborn child, it is advisable not to use cannabis during pregnancy, until there has been some clinical evidence that it is safe to do so.

3.4 PSYCHOSIS OR SCHIZOPHRENIA

In as much cannabis has been effective in treating other mental health conditions, if the drug is abused or used in excess, it causes some mental disturbances. There is a strong perceived relationship between the use of cannabis and schizophrenia, and this has been proven over the years. If cannabis is used in excess, it affects the brain chemistry, disrupting chemical balances and therefore causing mental disorder. The abuse of cannabis has two possible effects on the mental stability. It will either (i) start a full range of schizophrenia-like symptoms in healthy individuals or (ii) for patients harbouring psychosis, it will exacerbate and trigger a relapse of mental disturbances. Dr Hiroshi Ujike, a clinical psychiatrist at Okayama University, Japan, led a study examining the possibility of cannabis causing schizophrenia or psychosis. The results of the study were published in the Journal Molecular Psychiatry, showed that the excess use of cannabis made patients more vulnerable to schizophrenia and triggered the conditions for those already harbouring the disease. Although cannabis can be used to manage other mental health illnesses such as dementia, it is not suitable to treat schizophrenia, as it makes the condition worse.

3.5 CHRONIC BRONCHITIS

Patients diagnosed with chronic bronchitis need to take extra caution when taking cannabis treatment, especially for those using the smoking method of ingestion. Smoking cannabis presents increased symptoms of bronchitis and inflammation of the central airways which can lead to a higher chance of developing respiratory infections such as pneumonia. However, there have been conflicting studies regarding the effects of cannabis on the respiratory system, with some studies showing that a low dose of THC may be beneficial to the lungs. THC, which is the main psychoactive component of cannabis, can act as a bronchodilator, increasing oxygen flow to the lungs, thereby increasing lung efficiency. Although THC cannabinoids are beneficial to the lungs, for patients diagnosed with bronchitis, they should take it with caution.

3.6 RISK OF MYOCARDIAL INFARCTION

Myocardial infarction is one of the scariest risks associated with cannabis intake. Myocardial infarction, commonly known at heart attack, is a condition whereby the heart muscle dies, due to one of the arteries or branches supplying oxygenated blood becoming suddenly blocked, starving the heart muscle of oxygen. The use of cannabis has been linked to the increase in vascular conditions such as heart attack, stroke and transient ischemic attack (TIA). Acute doses of cannabis can negatively affect the cardiovascular system, presenting symptoms such as an increase in heart rate, high blood pressure and postural hypertension. The Institute of Medicine (1999) reported that these cardiovascular effects are likely to affect the older generation more than younger people. In as much as the thought of heart attack might be frightening, the good news is that the risk is very minimal. However, extra caution must be taken during cannabis treatment.

3.7 RISK OF OVERDOSING CANNABIS OIL

Just like any other medications, an overdose might have harmful effects on the body. Although an extra dose of cannabis taken might not be dangerous to cause any shut down in your body system, it can cause negative side effects and make you feel anxious and disoriented. To find the right dose, start with the lowest dose and increase gradually until you find the appropriate dose that your body tolerates. Remember dosages can vary with individuals. A dose can influence one person and might not influence another. Therefore, never use another person's dosage instructions.

3.8 DEPRESSION AND IRRITABILITY

Cannabinoids stimulate receptor sites CB1 and CB2 in the brain, which have a wide range of effects on mood, thoughts and feelings. When taking larger doses of cannabis oil, you can have side effects that are mood-related such as anxiety, depression and irritability. If experiencing these side effects, there isn't much that can be done except to keep yourself comfortable and ensure that you are well hydrated. These side effects can happen whilst you are on medical cannabis treatment and can also happen when coming off the treatment. Some scientists suggest increasing the amount of CBD oil being used whilst reducing THC at the same time, to counteract these side effects. Other cannabis users have claimed that the smell of rosemary flowers reduces the effects of inhaled cannabis. Therefore, a few drops of rosemary are worth a try. The *sativa* strain can make some people agitated, whilst the *Indica* has a calming effect and is better with anxiety disorders. Another side effect of cannabis is to re-surface one's buried psycho elements, trauma and emotions. All these side effects can bring undesired results, but they can be reduced with medication and a healthy organic diet.

4

SOURCES AND STORAGE OF CANNABIS OIL

4.1 HOW TO GET OIL IN THE UK

One of the biggest challenges for patients who wish to try cannabis treatment in the UK is how to obtain the oil, considering its legal status. Although cannabis oil has been legalised in some countries like the USA, it remains an illegal substance in the UK. However, there are weaker strains of cannabis such as CBD that can be available to purchase online in the UK. CBD oil has a reduced strength, with a lower ratio and is not strong enough to attack several diseases.

Apart from growing your own cannabis, it is difficult to acquire the best grade of cannabis and be self-sufficient with your own medicines. However, for UK residents, this might not be the best option in view of the legal status of cannabis. Most patients are currently using the Internet to source the full spectrum of both THC and CBD, which comes with its own challenges too. The cost of cannabinoids is expensive, from obtaining the raw materials to the processing and finally the finished product. Purchasing cannabis online can be prone to fraud and bogus sellers, and therefore, there is a need to be extra careful and take extra precaution. If you become a victim to fraud, there are no legal grounds to raise your case since cannabis is an unlegalized substance. Therefore, it is important to be extra vigilant.

4.2 TOP TIPS WHEN PURCHASING CANNABIS ONLINE

1. Do thorough research before purchasing the oil, ensuring the source of the oil is legitimate. Reviews will be the best tool to obtain information about the supplier and their product. Check for reviews

and seek recommendations from other patients who have bought the oil from the same buyer.

2. If possible, always look for sellers in your geographical region. If in Europe, try and buy from a European supplier. This will enable you to consider the applicable customs and border control, because customs have the right to seize any medical grade cannabis.

3. Avoid purchasing any oil from social media, as there are high chances of buying bogus oil. Social media such as Facebook and Instagram can harbour fraudsters as these platforms do not have tighter identification checks when setting an account with them.

4. To get all your questions answered, always ask for a phone call before purchasing. It would be more helpful if you request a Skype call or any other video call, to enable you to ask questions and judge their responses.

5. It is always important to check that the cannabis you are purchasing is from a genuine manufacturer with a valid test certificate. To prove the manufacturer is genuine, they must produce

a valid test certificate known as the HPCL test certificate. HPCL results provide information on the ratios and percentages of cannabinoids. If the supplier has the test done, then it's likely to be a genuine manufacturer, because the HPCL is an expensive test to do, and only genuine producers are likely to take the test. Having said that, you will still need to be careful because these HPCL results can be photo-shopped.

6. Don't send payment until you are satisfied with all the checks and are convinced that the supplier is genuine. Expect to pay approximately £50 per one gram of medical grade cannabis. The price of cannabis depends on the purity and quality, and in most countries where it is not yet legalised, patients obtain it through importation which makes it expensive. When making payment, never use cash services such as Western Union or MoneyGram, as this is the major indicator that the supplier is not genuine and is a fraudster.

7. Always ask for a sample to establish the authenticity of the products. However, not all suppliers can offer samples as this option is open to abuse. If

you get a sample, ensure there is THC and CBD in the oil, because these cannabinoids effectively work together, and for tougher diseases, a strain with a high THC content would be better.

4.3 HOW TO STORE CANNABIS

It is essential to store cannabis correctly because cannabinoids degrade when exposed to extreme conditions such as temperature, light and oxygen. These conditions affect the cannabis in different ways depending on whether it's the finished product cannabis oil or the raw cannabis herb. Refrigerating cannabis oil would be ideal because it will have a longer shelf life and improved quality. Cannabis oil can also be frozen for longer term storage and will maintain its potency and freshness for longer. The best way to freeze cannabis oil is to pack it into ice cube trays and put them into the freezer. All cannabis-infused products, including the oil, should be kept in a cool dark place and be sealed to avoid the exposure of light and oxygen because the light will degrade the cannabis trichomes.

Unlike cannabis oil, the storing of raw cannabis herb in the freezer or fridge has been controversial, with some arguing that exposing the herb to very cold temperatures will suck out the moisture and rupture the resin glands, resulting in less potent cannabis. It is also argued that the refrigerator is not the best storage place for the herb because of the temperature fluctuations that happen when the fridge is opened and closed frequently, therefore decreasing the herb's survival time.

Another important factor to consider when storing raw cannabis is the exposure to light and oxygen. Always store the herb in a cool dark place, and in airtight containers. Airtight glass containers are the best storage material for cannabis herb because they are impermeable, therefore no excess oxygen or moisture will get into the container. Avoid the use of plastic containers because the chemical in the plastic may alter the taste and aroma of the cannabis after some time. Dark coloured or opaque jars are effective in reducing the light exposure and thereby maintain the potency of THC-containing resin glands that are crucial in the treatment of diseases.

Another alternative option to airtight glass containers is CVault storage containers which are great for maintaining the ideal humidity of the herb. Excessive moisture can affect the herb and it will get mouldy. Therefore, it's important to maintain the right humidity which is about 65% on average. These CVault storage containers come with humidity packs and are made of food grade stainless steel. Although these containers are costlier than glass jars, they are the best option in ensuring desirable humidity, and preserve the herb throughout its shelf life. Another option is vacuum sealing, which is ideal for storing the herb for a longer time. Vacuum sealers eliminate all the air from the bag, which will cause the herb to degrade. Therefore, they are the perfect choice for long-term storage. These vacuum sealing bags are widely available for purchase online.

5

HOW TO MAKE YOUR OWN CANNABIS OIL

5.1 OVERVIEW

Making your own cannabis oil at home is another option to supply your own stock. To do this, you need to purchase raw cannabis and then make your own medicinal cannabis oil at home. This option will enable you to get the best quality oil known as full extract cannabis oil (FECO) and eliminate the risk of buying and using the bogus oils that are currently on the market. There are several methods for the preparation of cannabis, following the well-known method by Rick Simpson, who introduced the preparation of cannabis oil using naphtha and petroleum-ether as solvents. New recipes and ideas continue to spring up, with more emphasis on the type of solvent used in the preparation of cannabis oil, encouraging safer and organic solvents such as olive oil. Although there are various methods of preparation of cannabis oil, only one method will be outlined in this book, which is an easy and popular method of preparing the oil at home using a rice cooker. This process is very easy and quick, and it enables you to extract all the chlorophyll, which is essential for healing.

5.2 MATERIALS AND EQUIPMENT NEEDED

1. <u>*One ounce of high-grade medical cannabis*</u>. The actual amount of raw cannabis you will need depends on the type of disease being treated. To treat most cancers, approximately 60g/ml of cannabis oil is needed and can be produced with raw cannabis weighing one pound or more. Always acquire very dry cannabis, and for every ounce of high-quality cannabis bud used, 3-5 grams of cannabis oil is produced. Organic cannabis is the best option for those with a weakened immune system, as they might be affected by any residual

pesticides and fertilisers that may still be present in the herb.

2. *99%–100% isopropyl alcohol or Everclear*. This will be the solvent used in the process of extraction. For a pound of raw cannabis, two gallons of solvent would be enough to produce 60g/ml of cannabis oil.

3. *Rice cooker*. Apart from the rice cooker, some patients are making the oil using a green oil machine, which is an herbal extraction device that quickly, safely and efficiently extracts the essential oils from the cannabis plant. However, a rice cooker still does the job.

4. *Mixing bowls*. A medium or large mixing bowl would be ideal.

5. *Cheesecloth/nylon stocking/coffee filters/mesh strainer*. Any of these would do. These are used in the straining process.

6. *Wooden spoon*. A medium or large wooden spoon would be ideal. Needed for mixing.

7. _Silicone scraper set_. This must be able to withstand very high temperatures, as the mixture can be very hot.

8. _Large bottles_. These are needed to hold the solvent oil mix. A couple of bottles would be enough.

9. _Measuring cups_. These can be stainless steel.

10. _Oral syringes/empty capsules_. 10ml or 20ml oral syringes which are sterile. Needed for measuring or storing the completed cannabis oil. Both are available for purchase from pharmacies and online.

11. _Cooking thermometer_. For measuring the temperature of the mixture to ensure that desired cooking is achieved.

12. _Fans or ventilation if indoors/fire extinguisher_. For keeping the area well ventilated to avoid explosions. The fire extinguisher is needed in case of an explosion.

13. _Safety masks/glasses_. These are very important to ensure safety when preparing the cannabis oil, Proper safety equipment minimises exposure to the solvent.

14. _Oven gloves_. High heat gloves are essential for handling very hot cooker pots to prevent burns and splashbacks.

15. _Storage dish_. For storing the mixture.

16. _Candle warmer_. Needed for evaporating the carbon dioxide from the oil.

17. _Olive oil/coconut oil_. Used as a carrier oil (optional).

5.3 PREPARING THE WORKSPACE – STEP 1

The first step is to clean the workspace, wiping all counter tops and ensuring that the room is well ventilated by opening the windows. Adequate ventilation will prevent explosions and ensure that there is a fire extinguisher within reach in the unlikely event of a fire explosion. Gather all the materials within reach, including the safety equipment.

5.4 EXTRACTING THE SOLVENT – STEP 2

At this stage, we are removing the liquid cannabis from the herb by mixing it with high proof alcohol. Solvent extraction is a method used to separate a substance from a mixture by dissolving the substance in a suitable solvent. At this stage, you should have established which type of solvent is safer to use. In this example, I have chosen an alcohol high proof solvent because it eliminates potential carcinogens and the alcohol burns off in the process, so is a good option. The process of extracting the solvent consist of four stages. (i) The first step is to place dry raw cannabis into a mixing bowl or container which is big enough to hold the mixture. (ii) Then pour the solvent (alcohol) into the bowl Pour just enough to cover the herb. (iii) Then mix the cannabis herb with alcohol, stirring the mixture using a wooden spoon for a few minutes. (iv) Lightly crush the cannabis material for another two or three minutes, allowing the cannabinoids to dissolve all the plant material into the solvent.

5.5 STRAINING THE MIXTURE – STEP 3

Now we are separating the plant material from the solvent, and you can use any of the following: cheesecloth, nylon stockings, mesh strainers or coffee filters. By straining the mixture, we are stripping the cannabis plant 80% of its THC and other cannabinoids, using the following three steps: (i) cover the measuring cup using a cheesecloth or any other straining material of your choice, then pour the mixture over the cheesecloth to strain the plant material from the mixture; (ii) repeat this process again to ensure that all the bits are separated, using a second container and a clean cheesecloth; (iii) squeeze the remaining liquid off the cheesecloth, and you have a mixture of solvent and extracted cannabis resin which is a liquid dark green in colour.

5.6 SECOND SOAK – STEP 4

This step is to extract the remaining cannabis from the plant following the first soak. This is a repeat of Step 2, and you will need to do the following: (i) take the strained plant material and empty it back into the mixing bowl; (ii) pour the alcohol solvent – just enough to cover the plant material; (iii) mix and lightly crush for a few minutes to get the rest of the THC out of the plant; (iv) repeat Step 3, straining all the plant material from the mixture to ensure a pure and a good quality oil.

5.7 SEPARATING CANNABIS FROM THE SOLVENT – STEP 5

At this stage, you would have produced a dark green-coloured liquid, which is a mixture of cannabinoids and the solvent. The next process is to separate the cannabinoid resin from the solvent, and this is done by heat. This is when you need to ensure that the environment is safe and there is enough ventilation to avoid risk of an explosion. It is also advisable to test the maximum temperature your rice cooker gets to, and this is done by adding water to the rice cooker and then check the water temperature when it has reached its boiling point. Separating cannabis from the solvent consists of the following five steps: (i) firstly, add the solvent oil mix into the rice cooker, filling it up to three-quarters full to avoid spillages; (ii) turn the rice cooker onto a high heat and leave the lid open; (iii) allow the mixture to boil and continue to add the remaining mixture when the level in the rice cooker drops, and continue this until all the mixture is in the rice cooker; (iv) when the oil has become thick and less runny, remove the rice cooker pot from the machine. Remember to use oven gloves when handling the hot pot and ensure the room is well ventilated because these fumes coming from the pot can be flammable; (v) using a silicone spatula, remove the cannabis oil from the rice cooker into a bowl, this will be a shiny black oil that gives a golden amber colour when spread.

5.8 DECARBOXYLATION OF THE OIL – STEP 6

De-carbing the oil means removing carbon dioxide from the oil, and this can be done by evaporation. To evaporate carbon dioxide, you need to place the container holding the oil on a gentle heating device such as a candle warmer until the mixture has no bubbles appearing on the surface of the oil. The heating process can last between 3–24 hours for carbon dioxide to completely evaporate from the oil. However, be careful about heating the oil needlessly longer, because the longer the oil is heated on a gentle heat, the more sedative it will become.

5.9 ADDING THE CANNABIS MIXTURE TO THE CARRIER OIL

After Step 6, the medicine will be ready for use. However, some prefer to add their cannabis oil into a carrier oil, therefore this stage is only optional. At this stage, the ready-to-use cannabis oil is added into a carrier oil of your choice such as coconut oil or olive oil. Then heat the mixture on a gentle heat for an hour, until all mixed up. Coconut oil is one of the simplest and healthiest options for carrier oil and it is widely used for medicinal cannabis consumption. Coconut oil improves the immune system and is beneficial for the digestive system too. Using coconut oil as a carrier oil has an advantage in that it assists the cannabis oil in metabolising and helps to speed up the onset of relief. The combination of cannabis and coconut oil produces a powerful remedy because it contains a few acids such as caprylic and lauric acids which have antifungal and bacterial properties. However, coconut oil is not for everybody. Some still prefer to take the cannabis oil without a carrier oil, which is still fine.

5.10 PACKAGING THE CANNABIS OIL

When all is done, whether you have used a carrier oil or not, the final step is to package the cannabis oil. There are various methods of packaging the oil, depending on the method of ingestion to be used. Finished oil can be put in syringes and be taken like any syrup medication, or it can be put into empty capsules and ingested as tablets. To store the oil in the syringe, ensure that the oil has cooled first and then suck it up into the syringe. If using a capsule, you can then add the required dose in each capsule.

6

SAFE AND UNSAFE SOLVENTS

6.1 SAFE AND UNSAFE SOLVENTS

Solvents are one of the essential requirements in the production of cannabis oil and there is a wide variety of solvents available on the market. The type of solvent used determines the overall quality of cannabis oil produced. Therefore, it is important to choose a safe and non-toxic type of solvent. Organic solvents are the best option, coconut oil and olive oil, because they do not cause any harm to the overall health of the human body. In addition to organic solvents, there are alcoholic-based solvents, which are safe to use, and include Everclear, Spirytus vodka, ethanol and butane. Everclear is widely used in most countries and has been deemed to be safe. However, it's not currently available on the UK market. Patients from the UK have the option to use Spirytus vodka, a 96% ABV which is made in Poland, and can be purchased in most Polish shops around the country.

Extreme caution needs to be taken when choosing the type of solvent, because these unsafe solvents can present with numerous health hazards such as damage to the nervous system, liver, kidney, respiratory and skin disorders. Other unsafe solvents, if taken in excess, can lead to loss of consciousness, therefore the choice of solvent is important in the production of cannabis oil. Avoiding unsafe solvents is important because the residual from solvents – although some are non-toxic, they can negatively affect the health, causing long-term effects such as headaches, throat irritation, fatigue and allergic skin reactions.

6.2 OLIVE OIL – SAFE SOLVENT

All the disadvantages of other solvents leave olive oil as the optimal choice for the solvent in the preparation of cannabis oil. One of the major advantages of using olive oil is that it is affordable and easy to obtain as it can be found easily in high street shops. Non-flammability is one of the key qualities found in olive oil that makes that makes it the best choice. Olive oil is not flammable – therefore there is less risk of a fire or an explosion, and unlike other solvents, it guarantees safety during the production of cannabis oil. The process of using olive oil as a solvent is slightly different to that discussed in the previous chapter, as you can heat the cannabis-olive oil mixture up to a maximum of 100 degrees Celsius by placing the jar containing the mixture in boiling water for an hour or two. Unlike other solvents, olive oil cannot evaporate, so there is a need to consume large amounts of the oil to get the required dose of cannabis oil and achieve the same therapeutic effects.

6.3 ETHANOL AND BUTANE – SAFE SOLVENTS

According to the analytical study which was done to compare various methods of preparing cannabis oil, ethanol has been selected as one of the best solvents for extraction. Ethanol is proven to perform better in extracting a wide range of cannabinoids and terpenes that are found in the cannabis plant and are essential in the healing process. Ethanol is one of the active ingredients in most alcoholic drinks, but it's used in its concentrated form during the cannabis extraction process. Ethanol has a huge potential for abuse, and therefore it is restricted in most countries, including the UK. Although ethanol is excellent in removing cannabinoids, it has the disadvantage of producing an unpleasant taste, due to the large amounts of chlorophyll extracted from the cannabis plant. Some patients prefer to remove this chlorophyll by filtering ethanol using charcoal, but then it removes a huge number of cannabinoids which are needed for treatment, and thereby causing an adverse effect.

Butane is another hydrocarbon solvent which is currently being used to extract cannabinoids. The major advantage of butane is its non-polarity nature, which allows the solvent to capture the desired cannabinoids and terpenes from the plant, without co-extracting the chlorophyll and plant metabolites which are essential for healing. Another positive factor is that butane has a low boiling point of 0.5 degrees Celsius, which enables an easier purge from the concentrate when the process ends, therefore producing a pure by-product. However, despite butane having a low boiling point, it is highly combustible and there have been some cases of explosion reported. Therefore, practice extra caution. Other options for safer solvents include propane and hexane, and these are also widely used in the extraction process.

6.4 NAPHTHA AND PETROLEUM ETHER – UNSAFE SOLVENTS

Naphtha and petroleum ether are similar products with different names and are both considered unsafe for human consumption – a perfect example of an unsafe solvent. Naphtha is deemed unsafe because its vapour can cause symptoms of intoxication and in worst scenarios, depress the central nervous system. Other negative effects of naphtha's exposure to the human body include muscle weakness, loss of appetite, dizziness and drowsiness and therefore it is considered an unsafe solvent. Both naphtha and petroleum ether are a combination of petroleum hydrocarbons (PHCs) which makes them highly flammable and with a high boiling point of up to 200 degrees Celsius, it's extremely volatile, thereby posing a high risk of explosion.

7

RECOMMENDED DOSAGES AND DELIVERY ROUTES

7.1 STARTING DOSES FOR BEGINNERS

Taking cannabis for the first time can be a challenge, as people react differently to cannabis treatment. When taking cannabis for the first time, it is essential to build your tolerance levels slowly over the first 30 days to prevent the effects of a 'high' or extreme tiredness. Start with a very small dose such as the size of half a grain of rice, three times a day for seven days, leaving a gap of eight hours in between doses so that you can monitor the effects of each dose before you increase the dose. Following a week of taking the smallest dose, you can then increase the dose by doubling it. Continue doubling the dose every four days until the target dose of 1g/ml per day is achieved.

The normal overall dose for most patients is 60g taken in consecutive days, and this is usually effective in killing most cancers. The time needed to achieve the targeted dose varies per individual, but the average is between three to five weeks. Once you get the highest dose levels without any challenges, then continue at this dose until treatment has been achieved. The maximum dose is equal to eight or nine drops taken three times a day. However, if struggling to reach this dose, and experiencing negative effects such as extreme tiredness, then slightly reduce the daytime dose to about five to six drops at a time and increase the bedtime dose accordingly.

Measuring the oil in drops may be a challenge and a daunting process. To ease the process, put the oil into a carrier oil and measure using a syringe. For example, using coconut oil as a carrier oil, use a 20ml syringe to draw the coconut oil and squeeze into a jar that is resting in hot water. Then inject 1ml of cannabis oil into the jar and mix thoroughly until a light to a dark green colour is achieved. This dilution gives a ratio of

1/20g cannabis oil per gram of mixed coconut oil, and the cannabinoids will be completely bonded with the coconut oil fats. This dilution almost nullifies any chance of an overdose, although an overdose is not acutely harmful but can present with negative effects, which can be uncomfortable.

7.2 BUILDING YOUR TOLERANCE LEVELS

Cannabis tolerance levels differ for every individual, with some patients only able to take one capsule in a day whilst others tolerate up to 12 capsules per day. There are two approaches that have been proven effective in establishing the tolerance levels. The first is to start by the smallest dose in a capsule with a ratio of 20:1 and give it two hours. If there are no adverse reactions within the two hours, take another dose and wait for two hours again. Repeat this process until feeling some effects, and this will be your tolerance level – you can then stop. By counting the number of dosages taken, you are then able to establish your perfect dosages to start with. When building the tolerance level, the size of the body or weight has no effect on the dosages, therefore don't alter your dosages according to weight – stick to recommended dosages. Always maintain a two-hour gap between doses, because the body takes between half an hour to two hours to metabolise the cannabis and give the body time to feel the effects of the oil.

The second approach is to build your tolerance levels in five dosage levels until you get the final dosage level where the cannabis concentration will be higher. **_Dosage level 1 (1:20)_** – this is like the first approach; take one capsule, wait 90 minutes while monitoring the effects, and then take another capsule. **_Dosage level 2 (1:10)_** – using a carrier oil of your choice, mix 10 g of that oil with 1g of cannabis extract oil. Then take one capsule daily and gradually increase the capsules until you reach your tolerance levels. **_Dosage level 3 (1:5)_** – in the third dosage level, mix 5g of the carrier oil with 1g of extract cannabis oil. Start with one capsule per day and increase to two capsules daily. **_Dosage level 4 (1:1)_** – at this level, the strength of the capsules is increasing; mixing 1g of carrier oil with 1g of cannabis extract oil. Like the other stages, take one capsule per day, working your way up to two capsules daily. Because this is a strong dose, it is recommended to take a half dose in the morning and the other half dose at bedtime. **_Dosage level 5(1:0)_** – this is the final dose level, and cannabis is ingested without any dilution. As usual, start with 1g per day, working up to 3g per day. These levels will help you build your tolerance levels, and you can stop at any level if you feel you can't push it anymore, and therefore this will be your tolerance level.

7.3 DOSAGES FOR CANCER PATIENTS

It takes an average of 60g of cannabis to kill most cancers. Please note that this is just a recommendation, so some patients may need more cannabis to complete their treatment. Each type of cancer has a different dosing advice; therefore, it is important to get the correct dosage information before commencing treatment. Treatment of cancer requires properly produced cannabis oil, from a high-quality bud of sleepy sedative strains of *Indica*. The strain contains more than 20% of THC content and approximately 30g of raw cannabis is needed to produce oil from it. As mentioned earlier, start with a lower dose and then build your tolerance levels until you reach a comfortable dose.

The correct dosages for cancer depend on the type of cancer. Therefore, here are suggested doses for the following three types: breast cancer, lung cancer and skin cancers. For lung cancer treatment, the suggested dose is 500mg of THC per day, and for more aggressive tumours, 4g taken daily is advisable. However, there have been different opinions on the correct dosage which is effective in destroying the lung tumour. Some researchers suggest that taking a low dose of 30-40mg per day is more effective than higher doses, and patients on these low doses felt as much pain relief as those on higher doses. However, others still argue that high doses such as 400mg-1000mg per day are an effective dose in fighting aggressive cancer cells.

Although cannabis has been found effective in the treatment of breast cancer, incorrect dosages may lead to the tumour growing instead. Therefore, it is very important to use the correct dosage. Breast cancer is grouped into four categories, and the dosages vary according to the type of breast cancer. These four categories are: (i) oestrogen receptor positive (ER+), or progesterone receptor positive (PR+); (ii)HER2-positive; (iii) triple-negative; and (iv) triple-positive. According to the research, PR+, HER2-positive and triple-negative breast cancers have responded well to cannabis treatment with a high THC-CBD ratio of approximately 4:1. However, this dosage is not recommended for oestrogen breast cancers as it can cultivate the growth of tumour cells. For ER+ and triple-positive breast cancers, a dosage with lower THC-CBD ratio would be ideal – a ratio as low as 1:1 or 1:3 is recommended.

The recommended dosages for patients with skin cancers is 4 – 5 grams of high-quality cannabis oil. The perfect way to administer cannabis oil for skin cancer patients is to apply it topically, and as close to the tumour as possible, especially the carcinoma and melanoma tumours. Always ensure good hygiene and apply the oil, then cover with a clean bandage. For the cannabis oil to achieve the desired results, change the dressing and apply fresh oil every three or four days. Although some patients prefer to ingest the cannabis orally, the topical delivery route has proven to be effective for most skin cancers.

Although there have been several testimonies on the success of cannabis on cancer treatment, there is not enough clinical evidence that can make it the prime choice for cancer treatment. The conventional treatments of cancer, which include surgery, chemotherapy and radiation, should be pursued first before considering cannabis treatment option. Some patients choose to take cannabis treatment parallel to chemotherapy so that it reduces the nasty side effects of chemotherapy drugs. Cannabinoids can also be used in the maintenance and prevention of further re-occurrence of tumour cells in the body, and to replenish the good cells damaged by radiotherapy and chemotherapy.

7.4 IMPORTANT LIFESTYLE AND DIETARY CHANGES

For cannabis treatment to work effectively, ensure you follow a healthy diet, which is important in the healing of cancer and many other diseases. Therefore, consider changing your diet to healthier options. Cancer cells struggle to develop in a highly oxygenated and alkaline environment, so start eating foods that are high in alkaline such as green leafy vegetables. Chlorophyll is known to be the best alkaline food, and plant protein is effective in fighting the development of cancer cells. Therefore, it is highly recommended to be integrated into your diet. Avoid foods that promote a growing environment for cancer cells, such as dairy and meat products, and stay away from foods that are rich in sugar. Too much sugar negatively affects the body in various ways, so replace the use of regular sugar with raw honey, coconut sugar and other natural sweeteners. Avoid any types of soda drink, as they can contain too much sugar, and replace these soda drinks with juices that have no added sugar or make your own juice or smoothie at home. The best smoothie that will help to increase your PH level is made of ⅓ of celery, ⅓ of apple and ⅓ carrots blended together. Eating many fruits and vegetables is always good practice and beneficial for the body. It is recommended to take the seeds of two apples taken daily to provide the body with the required dosages of B17, which is useful in the treatment of cancer.

Another parasite that continues to feed the cancer cells is smoking. The smoke from cigarettes has a deadly effect on cancer patients and mostly affects patients diagnosed with lung cancer. There is a huge campaign by the government to discourage smoking and to improve every individual's wellbeing. Therefore, for those struggling to stop smoking, visit your GP and get some help. Exercise is one of the key issues in maintaining a healthy wellbeing, and oxygenating your body helps to fight the cancer cells. According to some research, some cancer types are because of deprivation of oxygen in the body cells. It is therefore essential to maintain regular exercise, which helps the body to oxygenate your body cells and increases your white cell count. There are many exercises that can be done at home without going to the gym – therefore, no excuses! Another good exercise to do is a light bouncing on the trampoline for at least 20 minutes every day, or to take a walk 3–4 times a week as this will increase your oxygen intake.

7.5 MAINTENANCE DOSES

After completing the cannabis treatment, and being in complete remission, it is advisable to continue taking a very low dose known as the maintenance dose. This is a very low dose of about 5% of a gram and no more than 100mg of cannabis per day. The purpose of taking this maintenance dose is to prevent the re-occurrence of the disease and the dose has no psycho effects on it. Apart from prophylaxis, the maintenance dose is used to control chronic conditions such as multiple sclerosis, lupus, Alzheimer's disease and Parkinson's disease.

8

HOW TO ADMINISTER CANNABIS OIL

8.1 OVERVIEW

The routes of administration are the method in which cannabis oil enters the human body in the bloodstream. There are five known and commonly used methods of ingesting cannabis oil which are: oral, topical, rectal or vaginal delivery, sublingual and the inhalation method. All these delivery routes are effective, depending on the type of disease being treated. However, the oral route is the most popular.

8.2 INHALATION METHOD

There are three ways in which cannabis can be inhaled: by smoking, vaporisation and dabbing. The effects of inhalation can last up to two hours, and this method is preferred by patients who are keen to feel the effects of the cannabis as soon as possible. During the inhalation process, cannabinoids enter the bloodstream through the lungs and take effect immediately. Smoking cannabis is part of the inhalation process. Only dried cannabis flower can be smoked and can be done using hand pipes or water pipes. Smoking cannabis is not recommended due to the negative effects it poses on the lungs, and it is also open to abuse, as some will turn it into recreational use.

The other method of inhalation is the vaporisation method, which is a healthier option to smoking as it eliminates irritation to the lungs and throat. To vaporise cannabis oil, heat it up enough to activate the psychoactive ingredients. The heated oil will then release the vapour, which is then vaporised, and the ingredients are absorbed into the lungs and forwarded into the bloodstream. Be careful of overheating the oil as it can release harmful toxins that can cause unwanted effects. Vaporisation is a much more effective method of ingesting cannabis oil than smoking as it cleans the lungs out of phlegm. There are various types of vaporisers on the market, and some require the herb to be finely ground before they can be vaporised. To produce a good quality vapour, it is important to ensure that there is less moisture within the herb, so avoid packing it tightly in the vaporiser as this could block the production of vapour by hindering airflow. Blocking the airflow in the vaporiser causes the cannabis herb to be too hot to produce vapour and can even lead to combustion.

The third method of inhalation is known as dabbing and is a comparatively newer delivery option. This method is like vaporisation – you will need highly concentrated cannabis oil and place it on a heated nail to create vapour. The vapour is then inhaled using a dab ring, and the effect is much stronger than that of smoking or vaporisation. However, this method can be a bit complicated for beginners. Therefore, it is only recommended for users with experience.

8.3 ORAL METHOD

This is the most popular way of administering medicinal cannabis and can be taken in two ways: as edibles or ingestible oils. Cannabis taken orally takes a bit longer for the effects to be felt, but once they kick in, the effects are intense, with long-lasting relief. The oral route delivery is slower because cannabinoids need to pass through the digestive system first before they can enter the bloodstream. Edibles are food or drink that has been infused with cannabis such as cookies, brownies, coffee and tea. These edibles are recommended and most effective for patients diagnosed with internal tumours such as leukaemia. The ingestible oils are any concentrated cannabis oil which can be taken orally via syringes or capsules. This can be the oil that you can make at home or purchase from a supplier, and it is also highly effective for internal cancers.

8.4 RECTAL/VAGINAL DELIVERY METHOD

Delivering cannabis though this method means you must use suppositories. Suppositories are ovular capsules that are inserted totally or vaginally, and these can be made at home by mixing ½ gram of cannabis oil with 2 grams of cocoa butter and heating the mixture, mixing it thoroughly during the process. Then leave it to cool and form the suppositories. The completed suppositories can be stored in the refrigerator ready for use. Each suppository contains a half gram of cannabis per dose. The suppositories are bio-viable and only take 10-15 minutes to take effect. Once inserted, the capsules dissolve and cannabinoids are absorbed through the thin lining of the intestinal wall. This delivery method is effective in the treatment of colon cancer, bowel cancer and vaginal cancers, and the main advantage of using this route is that the cannabinoids go directly into the bloodstream, bypassing the liver.

8.5 TOPICAL DELIVERY METHOD

This is the application of cannabis-infused products directly on the skin. These products include body creams, bath salts, body lotions and oils, and it's the best localised treatment, which is effective in reducing inflammation, joint pain and sore muscles. It is advised to mix one gram of cannabis oil in every 16 ounces of cream or lotion. However, in some cases, you can apply the concentrated cannabis oil directly to the skin. This method is highly recommended for treating skin cancers and other skin diseases such as eczema and psoriasis and it nourishes and improves skin elasticity. The topical method does not cause a 'high' effect and the therapeutic benefits of the cannabinoids are gently absorbed into the skin.

8.6 SUBLINGUAL DELIVERY METHOD

This is the final method of delivering cannabis, which is not very popular. Cannabis-infused products such as sprays, tinctures, and dissolvable strips are placed under the tongue, and the cannabinoids enter the bloodstream through the mucous membranes in the mouth. There are various types of cannabis sublingual products on the market, including cannabis-infused gums, which are not chewable but can be placed under the tongue until they are dissolved, and all the cannabinoids are absorbed.

CONCLUSION

I hope this book has enabled you to have a basic background of this magnificent herb which has the potential to provide treatment to many diseases. The cannabis plant, with its major cannabinoids such as THC and CBD, has been used to produce different types of cannabis oils that are essential in the healing of diseases. Although cannabis has not yet been legalised in the United Kingdom, there is ongoing extensive research being done in the country, with the hope of it being legalised soon. Cannabis has been proven to heal or manage symptoms of many diseases – the exciting one being the treatment of cancer, which gives many patients hope in fighting this deadly disease.

It is possible to make your own cannabis oil at home, if you ensure maximum safety and follow the instructions given. One of the important factors in making your own cannabis is to ensure that you use safer solvents of extraction such as Everclear, ethanol and butane solvents. Dosages of cannabis oil vary according to the type of disease being treated. Therefore, it is essential to follow advises on dosages.

Thank you again for reading this book. I hope you have found it the information useful and wish you all the best in the treatment of your selves and your loved ones.

www.ingramcontent.com/pod-product-compliance
Lightning Source LLC
Chambersburg PA
CBHW031925240526
45464CB00022B/862